GROWING CANNABIS

HOW TO CULTIVATE AND MAKE YOUR OWN CANNABIS GARDEN

BY SMART READS

Free Audiobook

As a thank you for being a Smart Reader you can choose 2 FREE audiobooks from audible.com. Simply sign up for free by visiting www.audibletrial.com/Travis to get your books.

Visit:

www.smartreads.co/freebooks
to receive Smart Reads books for FREE

Check us out on Instagram:

www.instagram.com/smart_readers
@smart_readers

ABOUT SMARTREADS

Choose Smart Reads and get smart every time. Smart Reads sorts through all the best content and condenses the most helpful information into easily digestible chunks.

We design our books to be short, easy to read and highly informative. Leaving you with maximum understanding in the least amount of time.

Smart Reads aims to accelerate the spread of quality information so we've taken the copyright off everything we publish and donate our material directly to the public domain. You can read our uncopyright below.

We believe in paying it forward and donate 5% of our net sales to Pencils of Promise to build schools, train teachers and support child education.

To limit our footprint and restore forests around the globe we are planting a tree for every 10 hardcover books we sell.

Thanks for choosing Smart Reads and helping us help the planet.

Sincerely,

Travis & the Smart Reads Team

TABLE OF CONTENTS

INTRODUCTION

Just like all natural medication, cannabis or marijuana has its own history. It is useful to understand why some properties or compounds have been widely ignored, while some others have been further promoted.

Over the years, the use of cannabis and marijuana as medical drugs have grown and this book will explore the various illnesses and conditions where cannabis can be and has been used as a treatment as well as the cultivation opportunities that may be available.

In genera, cannabis has been found to assist with anxiety disorders, schizophrenia, epilepsy, anorexia, and even cancer, just to name a few. Recent discoveries regarding the potential healing properties of cannabis have brought this once illegal plant back into the spotlight, only this time it has come back with positive reviews.

More research and clinical trials are being conducted in an attempt to find out the full potential of medical marijuana/cannabis. At this point it seems as though it can help with a wide array of health conditions.

The cannabis industry is maturing and the demand for more technical knowledge is intensifying. Major growing companies are focusing on increasing their production volumes, and of course, cashing in on potential profits. Many growers, however, especially those who have benefitted from collaboration, who have experimented and also succeeded through their own trial and error, are now starting to share their knowledge of cannabis cultivation.

Before legalization, most growers, especially independent ones had to keep their activities discrete. Even basic cannabis cultivation techniques had to be hidden and the more complex ones remained secret.

For some readers the information in this book will be completely new. For others, some of the information will be familiar with some new extras. It is becoming plainly clear that cannabis can be a serious alternative to so many toxic chemical medications.

Please read on and enjoy.

CHAPTER 1: A BRIEF HISTORY

The cannabis plant is nothing new. In fact, it has been around and has been used in different ways, including medicinally, for thousands of years. For most Westerners, cannabis conjures up thoughts or images of people who only want to get high, mostly associating it with the 60's and 70's.

For the most part of the 20th Century, cannabis and marijuana were criminalized and illegal in many parts of the world, especially in western nations. Therefore, the general opinion of cannabis was a negative one. Before that, cannabis extract was a popular medicinal drug in the Americas in the 1800's. However, this popularity began to change around the early 1900's. In the 1920's, Mexican immigrants became associated with the recreational, smoked version of marijuana and this fuelled the anti-immigrant sentiment that began to be felt throughout the U.S. and moved it towards prohibition.

This continued and by the 1930's cannabis was banned in 24 states. The Federal Bureau of Narcotics, which had been recently set up, began a campaign against the drug. Newspaper articles fuelled the negative view of the plant. Headlines such as "Murder Weed Found Up and Down the Coast" and "Deadly

Marijuana Dope Plant Ready for Harvest that Means Enslavement of California Children" began to appear.

In 1937, the U.S. Congress passed the Marihuana Tax Act. This meant that marijuana was banned completely, with the exception of few medicinal purposes. During the Second World War, the U.S. government subsidized hemp and U.S. farmers grew around one million acres as part of that program.

This negative view of cannabis and the seemingly continual negative attention from the media created a negative smoke screen and prevented many from seeing the true potential of the plant. Of course, marijuana plants are able to produce a variation of drugs.

Often, people grapple with whether or not a certain drug should be available freely or be kept discrete. Of course, many drugs can be, and sometimes are, misused, leading people to believe the same about cannabis. The fact is, drugs of many kinds that are even legal can be misused and do cause damage to people. However, it is unfortunate that the cannabis plant has had such a poor reputation in the west in particular. This has not been the case in many eastern nations.

Cannabis has been used for thousands of years throughout different cultures for its legitimate medicinal powers. A few cannabis plant species exist and there are sub-species of those as well. Every species and sub-species contain variations of different properties and because of this, cannabis can be seen for what it is - a versatile plant with enormous medical potential.

Cannabis has leaves that can grow leaflets on them, usually about six or seven per leaf, and sometimes up to thirteen per leaf. The leaves are often used as tea based therapy in many cultures. Ancient cultures used cannabis for its healing assets, including the Chinese, the Egyptians, and the Greeks. When the leaves are crushed and used in a tea, it can be a useful painkiller and provide relief to people who are suffering.

Ancient history shows that Shennong, the Chinese Emperor who lived around 5,000 years ago, kept detailed records of the different medicinal uses of marijuana. The Emperor would frequently use them himself. The records contain claims that marijuana was used as a cure for such ailments as gout, malaria, and even mild amnesia.

Cannabis has had a connected history with India as well, and was referred to as "sacred grass" in ancient

Indian texts. The Indians used cannabis a lot, including for recreation.

Recreational cannabis use spread to Europe by 500 AD. Later, some of it was brought back from Egypt by Napoleon's troops. Hashish smoking was common in the Middle East. Hashish is smoked through a type of vaporizer or heated pipe called a "bong" and is usually a solid or powdered form of cannabis plant resin.

Hemp is another category of cannabis and it was used extensively throughout the ancient world and even the modern one. This use has continued throughout the ages in Asia, even today. Hemp contains high levels of protein and therefore, can be used for different food items and fiber products. Hemp is still cannabis, however, it doesn't contain the often-feared "high" element, or the psychoactive agents that other varieties may contain.

By the 15th and 16th Century, cannabis was brought to Spain and then America. The cannabis plant was cultivated extensively in America and the fiber used for everyday items like cloth, paper and rope. Both George Washington as well as Thomas Jefferson grew cannabis and it is known the paper that the American Declaration of Independence was written on by

Jefferson was made from cannabis. Even the very first American flag was woven from cannabis plant fibers.

Throughout the 18th and 19th Centuries, American pharmacies had cannabis listed under medication. They used it to help with the relief of arthritic pain, to suppress nausea as well as reduce the pain of childbirth.

Americans, in particular, musicians or show business individuals popularized its use and this led to recreational marijuana joints disguised as clubs. These were called "teapads" and sprouted in different places countrywide.

By the early 1950's, cannabis usage steadily increased once more, and once the hippie movement arrived, it fueled the use of cannabis further by the 60's. Cannabis became a symbol for non-conforming, American youths who were rebelling against their government.

U.S. Congress at this point decided to classify cannabis alongside other hard substances such as heroin, as a "Schedule 1" drug and it was officially considered a hard drug. Critics of this act believed that subsequent U.S. governments who applied it strictly then prompted a huge increase of arrests as well as an overpopulation of the prison system. Most of those arrested and imprisoned for possession were from certain ethnic minority groups like African Americans and Hispanics. Many of these people were innocent of any violent crimes.

Certain other governments such as the Mexican government, followed America in this regard and began to destroy all the cannabis plants throughout the country. This then opened the way for drug cartels in other places like Colombia to capitalize on these particular laws and intensify their operations even more, making their country one of the major cannabis suppliers.

In the 1990s, the state of California legalized cannabis for medical purposes only. Some other states followed this trend. There have been a few United States presidents that have used cannabis as well.

Marijuana even has its own day - April 20th, which is "International Marijuana Day." Twenty-three states in the US have now legalized the use of cannabis for medicinal purposes and a small number allow it for recreational purposes. In 2013, Uruguay was the first country in the world to fully legalize cannabis use. Other nations have decriminalized cannabis even for recreational purposes.

In Holland, coffee shops can sell soft drugs to customers, but no more than five grams of cannabis per person per day. All coffee shops must adhere to strict laws and adhere to the legal amount of soft drugs and the conditions in which they are sold and used. They cannot advertise drugs or sell them to under 18's.

In Ukraine, it is legal to possess up to 5 grams of cannabis. You can also cultivate it as long as it's no more than 10 plants. Buying and selling cannabis is illegal.

In Portugal in 2000, there were changes to the law which meant that consumption and /or possession of all illegal drugs found only in small quantities was decriminalized. This means that possession of personal quantities of drugs, including cannabis, is not a criminal offence.

Going by this, it seems it probably won't be too long before other countries begin the transition.

CHAPTER 2: MEDICINAL USES

For thousands of years, cannabis was used in traditional medicine throughout many parts of the world. Today, with advances made in scientific testing and clinical trials, medicinal applications used previously have now been verified and found to be true. Even more uses for the cannabis plant's healing properties are being identified as research continues.

Cannabis has historically been used for different physical and mental/emotional ailments. It was used as an effective pain reliever and can assist with conditions such as arthritis, anorexia, nausea, epilepsy, heart disease, and even labor pains during childbirth, just to name a few. More are mentioned below:

- Obesity
- Glaucoma
- Cancer
- Chronic pain
- Heart disease
- Multiple Sclerosis
- Osteoporosis
- Schizophrenia
- Anxiety and Stress
- Metabolic syndrome-related disorders

Cannabis also has the potential to help with the relief of certain symptoms of cancer and HIV. It has been found to be anti-tumoral and anti-cancerous, killing off cancer cells while leaving healthy cells intact. Cannabis has some potential in reducing cholesterol within the bloodstream and also helps reduce the fat deposits that might surround organs such as the liver. This can help those who suffer from type 2 diabetes.

In addition, THCV, which is one of the compounds found in certain cannabis strains, helps to increase insulin sensitivity and protect insulin-producing cells found in the human body. It does this by forming a protective layer. THCV also seems to increase productivity and longevity in cells that produce insulin.

Cannabis plants contain different compounds, some of which are very valuable for humans. CBD, for example, which is short for cannabidiol, is one of those compounds found in the well-known and once illicit cannabis, as well as the legal industrial component of cannabis, which is called hemp. It now seems like CBD has a lot to offer. The CBD compound has significant medical benefits without causing users to get "high." It is only in recent years that cannabis, CBD and THC, another cannabis compound, has seen positive media attention, and this attention has removed the stigma to a great extent.

Some compounds in cannabis have been found to suppress appetite (and are different to those that increase appetite and can be used to treat anorexia). These compounds are now being researched some more for their potential in managing obesity. Cannabinoids also possess muscle-relaxing properties. There are trials being conducted to discover if they might offer solutions for conditions like multiple sclerosis. They have already been found to have positive effects on people with certain types of epilepsy.

When you look at a cannabis bud you can see the resin. When examined microscopically, these resins tend to look like crystals and when heated or smoked, these crystals release certain compounds. Understanding the chemical composition of these compounds will reveal why cannabis is considered valuable. Two chemical categories of cannabis are Cannabinoids and Terpenoids.

Cannabinoids:
Cannabinoids are medicinal and psychoactive molecules. These give cannabis its potency and can be

addictive. They are usually acidic before they are broken down.

• Cannabidiol or CBD

This has been found useful with seizures and is used for conditions such as multiple sclerosis and epilepsy. CBD compounds are not psychoactive but they are calming. CBDs are used for the relief of stress and reduction of insomnia as well as diabetes.

• Tetrahydrocannabinol or THC

This compound in cannabis is a psychoactive cannabinoid. It has many healing properties including pain relief, reducing nausea (antiemetic) and helps with muscle spasticity.

• Cannabinol or CBN

When THC is heated, it produces the CBN compound. CBN, like CBD, can also help with sleep disorders like insomnia. It is a very strong sedative. It also contains antiemetic properties and therefore helps to curb nausea.

• Cannabigerol or CBG

CBG is a precursor to both CBD and THC. It is non-psychoactive (like CBD) and has a special characteristic that is that it's able to stimulate brain cell growth. Some scientists believe that, in order to achieve the full psychoactive effect during cannabis usage, CBG compounds must be present.

•   Cannabichromene or CBC
CBC is another non-psychoactive compound. It is effective in treating anxiety and stress-related conditions. It can also help with inflammation.

•   Terpenoids:
Terpindois are what give every cannabis species its own specific scent and flavor. Different cannabis species will have their own terpenoids.

•   B-Caryophyllene
This terpenoid contains antiseptic, antibacterial, and antifungal properties. It has a spicy kind of aroma that can be found in such plants as Thai basil, cloves, and black pepper.

•   Limonene
This is a terpenoid that emits a citrus scent. It contains anti-fungal properties. It is efficient in treating gastric reflux.

•   Terpinolene
This has a woody/smoky, earthy scent. For many centuries, it was used as an antiseptic and still is today.

- Myrcene

B-Myrcene can be found not only in cannabis but also in mangoes. Cannabis users will experience highs of greater intensity if they eat a mango before they use cannabis. These terpenoid activities are evident in the brain. They lower blood to brain barrier resistance and increase the maximum saturation of the brain's cannabinoid receptors.

- Linalool

Linalool is a terpenoid that can be found in other plants apart from cannabis. Plants such as rosewood, lavender, coriander, and birch contain it as well. It works as a painkiller and is a precursor in the production of Vitamin E. It also acts as an effective insecticide.

Cannabis Sativa varieties actually have the highest Terpinolene levels. In addition, they contain high levels of B-Myrcene. Meanwhile, Cannabis Indica species contain more Linalool, B-Caryophyllene and Limonene.

Considering all the compounds found in cannabis including those mentioned above, it is easy to see how its potential medicinal use should be further examined and tested. More research is needed to find out exactly how much medical potential cannabis actually has.

There are three main ways that cannabis is consumed:

1. Through Inhalation
This is usually the most common way and also the most potent. There is more than one way to inhale cannabis. It can be through rolls, pipes or often today, vaporizers.

2. Topical Application
These are usually for more localized pain whereby the cannabis oil is placed in a carrier oil (almond or coconut oil, for example) and then it can be topically applied.

3. Through Ingestion
Cannabis can also be ingested orally in the form of edibles, teas, tinctures, oils or capsules. It will take longer for the effects to be felt but they are stronger and last for longer periods than they do with inhalation. The average time is about 30 minutes after ingesting cannabis that people report feeling its effects. During the digestion process, cannabinoids undergo a chemical transformation and this makes them stronger. The only issue with taking cannabis orally is that it is a little more difficult to ascertain the

exact amount of the dosage due to the increase in time effect onset.

CHAPTER 3: LEGALIZATION

The law of the area where you live in governs cannabis usage. Usually, the law would govern whether it is legal for general purposes, medical or recreational. Anybody who grows or uses cannabis must know the laws that refer to cannabis usage in their state or area. These laws can be easily found and are in the public domain.

Globally, some nations are more liberal when it comes to marijuana, while others are not, as briefly mentioned before. Americans might be surprised to learn that cannabis is decriminalized in some other countries and has been for some time now.

This means that using it or possessing it is not seen as a criminal offense. In some places marijuana can be legally sold in coffee shops and other places as long as it is only a certain amount per person per day. Holland is one of those places. However, it is actually illegal to produce, import or export drugs, including cannabis, into Holland.

In Ukraine, it is legal to possess up to 5 grams of cannabis. You can also cultivate it as long as it's no more than 10 plants. Buying and selling cannabis is illegal.

In other places, cannabis possession can bring with it heavy fines or imprisonment. All travelers are urged to check the websites of individual governments before embarking on an overseas journey, not only for drug information, but also for anything else that is necessary to know.

In the United States, four states have decriminalized small quantities of cannabis use and possession. Washington State and Colorado are two of them. In 2013, Colorado became the first fully regulated market for recreational cannabis for adults in the world. Uruguay was the first country to fully legalize cannabis production, sale and distribution.

In the U.S., the laws governing cannabis use differ from state to state. Other states have legalized psychoactive or non-psychoactive medical cannabis. A total of 23 states and Washington DC have legalized cannabis usage in some form, but there are still about 22 states and 2 territories that totally prohibit the use of cannabis for any reason.

The University of Mississippi has been and continues to be, the official cannabis grower in the U.S. since 1968. As the laws around cannabis use have been changing lately, there is a growing demand for it both medically and recreationally. Someone must fill this supply gap. The estimated economic effect of cannabis being fully legalized throughout the U.S. is about USD $40 to $60 billion per annum. This is an industry that is gaining momentum and more and more farmers will be needed to keep up with demand.

CHAPTER 4: DIFFERENT TYPES OF CANNABIS

A cannabis plant can be female or male therefore it is referred to as being dioecious. Some of them are both and are referred to as being hermaphrodite. Male cannabis plants pollinate female plants. Once the female plant has been pollinated, it will develop its seeds, which will mature, then ripen, and eventually fall off the plant.

The Sativa cannabis species is found in abundance in the more tropical regions of the world such as the Caribbean, parts of Africa, the Middle East and also Mexico. The main characteristic of the sativa plant is the leaf shape. It has leaves that are long and thin. The cannabis Sativa plants are also much taller in height and take a bit longer to grow compared to other cannabis species. This is probably because they have adapted to their environments.

In the more temperate or colder regions of the world such as Europe, Northern United States, and Canada, cannabis Indica species is a lot more common. These plants have broader leaves and are shorter than the Sativa species. Cannabis Indica also have shorter maturity periods.

Another cannabis strain is the Ruderalis. This has much lower THC amounts and is also the least popular. The Ruderalis cannabis is mostly used for making fabric for clothing, shoes, and ropes. Other hybrids of cannabis exist such as Skunk, Bud, Orange, Northern Lights, and Blueberry.

No matter what the cannabis strain, they all contain these unique compounds called cannabinoids.

These can be broken down into two categories – cannabinoids and terpenoids. Both cannabis Indica and Sativa have chemical compositions that make them unique. The compounds which each variety contains will determine what uses would be best for each plant species.

The different compounds will also determine the cannabis scent as well as the various uses, either medicinal or not, that they can be used for. Higher levels of just one compound in cannabis Sativa could cause it to have properties of a psychedelic nature, and another cannabinoid in cannabis Indica helps to make it more calming.

CHAPTER 5: CANNABIS – AN ANATOMY

It is necessary for those using cannabis or those who may wish to grow it (only if it is legal in their area) to know about and understand the different parts of the cannabis plant. This will help with cultivating a higher quality crop.

It is the female plants that produce a flower cluster that secretes resin. They are then trimmed into the buds, which are generally the most sought after, higher priced, and the most valuable part of the cannabis plant. The male cannabis plants will pollinate the female plants, which will initiate the seed production. It seems simple at first, however, there is more to it.

Female cannabis plants that are un-pollinated can still produce buds. Not only that, but the cannabinoid in the bud resin from an un-pollinated, seedless female plant is quite rich. Due to this, the majority of growers prefer to grow seedless, female plants exclusively. Ultimately, this will translate into more profit because the more seedless, female plants a grower has, the more flowers there will be. More flowers will then produce more buds and there you have it – more money for the growers.

Cannabis being a plant also has certain features similar to other flowering type plants. However, its other physical characteristics are very different. Cannabis, for example, grows on very long stems, its leaves like small fans extending out from the nodes.

Often, there is a cluster from where female flowers bloom. These are called colas. The major one is usually the first one to appear and can be seen at the top of the cannabis plant. It is also often the largest one and sometimes called the apex cola. On the plant nodes there will be smaller colas that will begin to grow after the main one has appeared.

Once you know what you're looking for, you will be able to see that the female plant flower is not a single cluster but has quite a few. These calyxes will appear in different sizes, shapes, and colors. They secrete cannabinoids that the end user will enjoy through certain glands called the trichomes.

From the calyx there will be small hair-like strands that spring out and are a vibrant orange-yellow-red color. They are called pistils and when they initially appear they will be white and later their color darkens to yellow, red, orange, amber, or brown. These colors help to make the buds of the cannabis plant more appealing to the eye.

Pistils have a major role in female reproduction as they receive pollen from the male plants. They don't have any effect on the buds in terms of their flavor or their potency.

The cannabis flowers, leaves, trims, stem tips and hash are all used to make certain products such as oil. The main ingredient is the leaf but other parts of the cannabis plant when used, are believed to add an even wider spectrum to the oil.

CHAPTER 6: CULTIVATION

Quite often, commercial cannabis growers will cultivate the plants indoors and under controlled environments. Desired results can be more easily achieved in these types of environments and the plants will be easier to harvest and produce better quality products.

Controlled Cannabis Growing Environments
Growing cannabis plants inside a carefully controlled space or environment is becoming a popular farming technique. These areas are called grow rooms and are enclosed spaces that are sterile and devoted to cannabis cultivation. It is a good way to use a limited amount of space as well as increase the chances of a good yield. When cannabis plants are grown in these controlled environments, it will allow the growers certain advantages, primarily they can have a lot more control over the management of their crops' lifecycles along with the product quality as well. This will lead to the production of similarly good quality products, as the crops are all grown in the same simulated environmental state.

Disease control is another advantage when planting in grow rooms. If, in any situation, there is any kind of outbreak, it is much easier and quicker to find the problematic plant and eliminate it so they do not spread any infection to other plants. This is much harder to do in an outdoor growing environment.

Growing Environment: The cannabis farmers aim is to recreate every element of the outdoor natural environment within a grow room. Specific types of equipment and some technical implementations are essential to creating a proper grow room.

- **Space and Reflective Coverings:** The design of a cannabis grow room needs to be thought out well. It is not something that can be thrown together overnight. First, the space that is needed per plant is around one square meter. Knowing this it can be easier to estimate how much space will be needed and/or how many plants can be fitted into a particular space.

Grow room sizes might range from a large garage or basement area to a small cupboard space. The only thing necessary is for the space to be enclosed and that the right amount of cannabis plants are cultivated per meter so as to avoid overcrowding. If overcrowding occurs it can stunt the plant growth.

Grow room space that is underutilized should be reviewed, in particular when a grower is planting cannabis for commercial purposes. If the space seems too big then it might be necessary to increase the seedling numbers that are planted.

A reflective material should be covering the ceiling and walls of grow rooms. Plastic can be utilized for this. Painting the walls white is also a good idea as this will increase and conserve light within grow rooms. The correct lighting is of utmost importance and will make a big difference in not only the quality of the plants but also the quantity. Reflective ceiling and walls will make sure that light isn't wasted. It will be reflected back onto the plants thus helping them to grow as high as they can.

•	**Lighting and Reflective Hoods:** As mentioned in the paragraph above, the right type of lighting and regulation of the lighting is of utmost importance for indoor cannabis growing. More buds will be produced if the lighting is consistent and better quality. It will not work with regular halogen, incandescent light bulbs commonly used in homes. Fluorescent lighting can be utilized for growing the seedlings and also clones, however, the lighting must be changed as the cannabis plants start to grow older. It must be an HID (High-Intensity Discharge) light. These lights supply the correct type of heat and illumination to help cannabis plants grow well into their flowering and also vegetative stages.

HIDs or High-Pressure Sodium and Metal Halide lighting can be 400, 600 or 1,000 watts. As usual, the light emitted will be much brighter depending on the wattage. The higher the wattage the more electricity will be needed to power the lights. Metal Halide lights emit lighting that is similar to sunlight. For this reason they are preferred for the vegetation phases. High-Pressure Sodium light bulbs emit a yellow-orange light that is more suited for the flowering stage. Growers will usually use a combination of both light types in grow rooms but if a grower decides to use only one type then the High-Pressure Sodium is the way to go.

Higher wattage will bring higher lumen. Metal Halide lights/lamps generally have lower levels of lumen compared to the High-Pressure Sodium Lamps of similar wattage. This is why High-Pressure sodium lamps are brighter than the Metal Halide lamps with similar wattage.

The type of lighting, as well as the quantity and quality of bulbs needed for the cannabis plants will be determined by the grow room size. For smaller rooms, lower wattage light bulbs can be utilized and bigger ones in bigger rooms. Professional growers are able to produce one pound of buds for every 1000-watt bulb that is used. Placing reflective hoods over HID lights in grow rooms will optimize light consumption and ensure that the light will reflect onto the cannabis plants directly.

In order to properly mimic sunlight, the bulbs in growing rooms must be suitable. They will emit quite a lot of heat. This heat will intensify during the summer months when it's also hot outside. For this reason, some indoor growers like to use basements as grow rooms, especially when the houses that they're in have no air-conditioning. A basement's location tends to keep it cooler so it's perfect for limiting heat.

• **Thermometers**: Cannabis grow rooms will need temperatures of between 70- 85°F (or 20 to 30°C). This is the ideal temperature. The grow room lights will produce heat and the vents and fans will also affect the room temperature. Depending on the season, the temperature in the grow room will increase or drop. Carefully decreasing or increasing air coming in through the fans will help to regulate the temperature. In very hot climates air-conditioners can be used to reduce the extreme heat in the summer months.

- **Growing Methods:** There are plenty of choices available for those who want to select a growing method for cannabis. The main thing is to make sure that the growing mediums are light grow mixes with textured, soft grains that can hold water as well as drain off any excess. A lot of growers are now using soil-less mixes. Potting soil can also be very good for this. Both potting soil and grow mix are easy to find.

When it comes to fertilizers, they are added when using soil mixes, however, soilless mixes don't come with fertilizers. Purchasing soil-less mixes or plain soil mixes is a better idea. You can then fertilize them with the perfect amount for cannabis plant growing. Fertilizers can be mixed in with soilless mixes before the planting. They can also be added in a liquid form later on when watering the plant.

Using chemical fertilizers has become more common as they are easy to use and only require basic knowledge. They don't need any complex mixing techniques. Chemical fertilizers basically contain the NPK combination, which is Nitrogen, Potassium, and Phosphorous. Cannabis plants thrive on these minerals and other secondary trace nutrients. Organic fertilizers are harder to understand, however, cannabis growers who use them say that the final product is tastier and cleaner.

All fertilizers must be utilized according to the instructions. Some people are tempted to over fertilize. Around two weeks before buds are harvested, which is close to the last stage of the cannabis plants' life, no fertilization is necessary. If fertilizer is added during this stage, bud quality will be affected.

Soil mixes tend to be sterilized before being packaged. This ensures they are free of any disease-causing microorganisms or pathogens. This gives it an advantage over regular garden soil.

- **Wiring**: Grow rooms must be electrically wired for powering the lights, timers, fans, and other types of equipment that might be needed in the rooms. Cannabis grown in houses will often be done in enclosed rooms. For this reason, it is of utmost importance to strictly adhere to safety standards when wiring is done for a grow room.

The lights used in cannabis grow rooms are higher wattage lights therefore a different circuit should be made for grow rooms separate to the house wiring. Of course, the electric bills will increase.

Any naked wires must be appropriately covered in these rooms because they are warmer and tend to be isolated.

- **Watering**: Cannabis plants need generous amounts of good quality water. Most tap water will do. Water from wells can sometimes contain salt so for this reason it's best to avoid it if possible. Water pH levels of 6-8 should be fine for cannabis cultivation.

In addition to the actual water itself, suitable drainage channels are also needed. Proper plumbing needs to be developed in grow rooms to ensure that easy drainage can occur. In some cases, drainage pipes may not be installed. In these cases, troughs or trays can be put in place to collect any water run-off. Watering the plants has to be done evenly and slowly around the plant roots. This is to ensure the growing medium doesn't harden and become a solid piece, leaving spaces around pots where the water can easily escape.

As they grow and mature, cannabis plants will need more water. Soil-less mixes also increase the plants' need for water. Usually, the cannabis plants must be watered every second day. They must be watered regularly or they can become dehydrated which will lead to leaf and branch drooping.

The stems and leaves must also be sprayed with water. This is to imitate normal rainfall in a natural environment. The best time to do the misting is just before the grow room lights are switched off. This way the water droplets don't evaporate too quickly. Misting will help keep the stems and leaves moist and also remove any dust that may have settled on their surface getting into the leaves' pores.

When fertilizers or other chemicals are used, more water will be necessary, as they will cause a salt build-up to occur. Using around three times the water than usual can solve this problem. The water helps to clean this out when it drains it from the bottom.

•	**Proper Ventilation:** Air ventilation is absolutely necessary and something that mustn't be compromised in grow rooms. All plants need constant carbon dioxide. Air must be supplied. When the air becomes stale, removal will be necessary. In order to do this, two main vents would be needed. One to allow fresh air to enter and another exhaust vent for expelling stale air. Fans can also be attached to vents that will help with drawing in fresh air or expelling stale air.

Suitable ventilation will also help curb any plant odors. Sometimes they can become so strong that even the grow room vents cannot curb them. If this is the case, ozone generators could be used. They are effective but also expensive and may require some additional construction. Carbon filters can be an excellent alternative. They can be attached to exhaust fans to curb any odors. They filter odors through charcoal in their filters as they expel the air. They are much easier to install and use than the ozone generators.

The fans are necessary as they are a replacement for wind, which stirs the leaves and the stalks to make them stronger. It also helps to keep dust and bugs at bay. The fans will make quite a bit of noise, however, even if there is thick insulation around the grow room.

Due to this, and the odors that will eventuate, it will be necessary for growers to then carefully think about the location of their grow rooms. Locations such as house basements, garages, or backrooms can be used but again the individual must think about everything mentioned above, including the noise factor. For those who can afford to, changing the grow room design might be an alternative. Double insulation on walls and special types of filter boxes will reduce noise and odors. Baffle boxes could also be fitted onto fans to muffle any excessive noise.

- **Timers**: Timers will be necessary to help turn lights on and off and keep pumps going during the plants' lifecycles as well as controlling the vents and fans. These would obviously be electronic and digital timers. Several types of timers can be used but one thing to keep in mind is that the timer selected should be easy to use and easily replaceable should it wear out – and it will.

- **Disease and Pests**: Poor ventilation, temperature, and humidity will encourage spider mite growth. Temperatures at 75 degrees Fahrenheit and oscillating fans will assist in warding off insects and other pests. When dealing with an insect infestation, and it will likely occur, farmers have found that spraying the cannabis leaves (both front and back) with water and dish soap, is effective, especially for insects like spider mites. Pesticides also work; however, it is best to avoid them due to the chemicals they contain. If using pesticides, they are never to be sprayed on the buds. Introducing more natural pest control such as ladybugs is one way to do this. Growing certain other plants between them also helps.

Pest control is something outdoor cannabis growers have to deal with effectively in a manner that will not hurt the plants. Whether its insects, birds, mammals or even humans, cultivated plants often seem to be targets. Certain pests seem to like the taste of raw cannabis. If this is left unchecked, infestations could ruin the crop. However, pesticides or other harsh chemicals can also be harmful to the plants. So, what can be done in the outdoors?

Ensure the soil or fertilizer is sterilized so that no eggs or larvae are present. Growing companion plants that are natural repellents in between, such as basil, mint, geraniums or marigolds, is a good way of keeping pests and predators away.

- **Mold**: This can be a problem when cultivating cannabis. Both black and white mold infestations can be challenging if they are not handled immediately and correctly. The white mold comes from high humidity and is powdery in texture. It also comes from spaying the cannabis leaves with water, which is something unavoidable. Black or grey mold could appear in later stages of cannabis plant development when flower clusters are thicker. It can also come about due to cut or damaged stalks. It is always necessary to check for mold.

- **Caution**: Grow rooms should be kept very clean, sterile even, and also clutter free in order to prevent disease or infestation. The only items or equipment that should be in grow rooms are those that are frequently used to maintain the plants. Anything used in the grow rooms that is removed for use elsewhere must be sterilized again before bringing it back in. Unsterilized equipment has the potential to introduce diseases. Even any new equipment must be sterilized and cleaned carefully before going into grow rooms.

Using only specific clothes for the grow rooms is a good idea. Carpets are not necessary in a grow room especially if they become wet, as the dampness will create the potential for harmful insects or microorganisms. Grow rooms are best without carpeting. They should be thoroughly cleaned with light bleach water. However, in the case of carpets having to remain, for whatever reason, they must be cleaned, then sterilized and covered properly with plastic that can stop water dropping onto them and causing dampness.

When the cannabis plants start shedding their leaves, the water will begin to run off from the bottom of the planting pots and mustn't be allowed to accumulate in a grow room. The humidity levels in grow rooms should be between 40 – 60%. In dry environments, humidifiers can be utilized, or in opposite environments dehumidifiers can be utilized.

CHAPTER 7: SPECIES DETERMINATION

Indoor growers prefer cannabis Indica for a few different reasons. Firstly, its growing period is shorter and quicker than the other species of cannabis. Due to this it can be cultivated a few times within one growing period. Having a shorter growing period is also better as it reduces the risks of disease exposure.

The Seeds

In certain other countries that have no legal restriction on the use of cannabis, several different seed companies exist that are retailers for cannabis seeds. Online suppliers are also available, however, the most important thing is making sure the company is reputable. Some companies will not ship to the U.S. It is important to do your own research.

As with most retail products the prices will vary with each company. Prices, however, are not necessarily a guarantee of quality. It is the reputation of the company that will better indicate whether the seeds will be good quality. If cannabis cultivation is legal in your area, local growers will also supply good quality seeds.

Germinating Cannabis Seeds

Cannabis seeds are quite small. In fact, they are about the same size as a matchstick head. Sprouting the cannabis seeds is the first step to growing cannabis.

There are different ways of doing this:
1: Seeds can be placed in water for 24 hours after which they should be examined. What you are looking for is a tiny, white root pushing out of one end. It will mean the plant has sprouted. At this stage the water should be drained and any seeds, which didn't sprout, discarded. Once this is done, the healthy seeds will be transferred to a growing medium.

2: Using a kitchen tray and some kitchen towels layered on top of one another (paper ones), moisten the towels with water. This will create another sprouting medium. The seeds should then be distributed evenly (not clustered close together) around the tray, which is then placed onto an elevated surface. Leave until the seeds sprout. Many growers work with this method.

3: A tray or soil bed can be used instead of paper towels. Seeds are placed in the soil half to one inch deep and allowed to sprout.

No matter what the method, there are some things that must be noted. Firstly, the tray holding the seeds must never be left on the floor. Cold temperatures from the ground could inhibit seed growth. As mentioned, an elevated surface is best.

Secondly, the seeds can be covered with a humidity or moisture dome, which is sold in the gardening section of larger retail stores. The trays that are used can also be bought from the same stores and because they are made of plastic they prevent moisture escaping. They will also allow light to get into the plants and protect the seedlings, which are very delicate at this stage, from any harsher environmental conditions. They also allow growers to watch as the plants grow. It only takes around 3 or 4 days for the seeds to sprout.

Alternative Sprouting Method – Clones/Cuttings
Cannabis plants can also be grown by using clones or cuttings (clippings) from mature plants. This is the way many plants can be grown and cannabis is no different. Each clone will be identical genetically to the "parent" plant, the one it was taken from originally.

As already mentioned briefly, it is the unpollinated female plants which are seedless that will yield more economic value because of the buds they have. Therefore, feminized cannabis seeds are more sought after. Many times, clones or cuttings are taken from these female plants, which will optimize the growing time and therefore the profit.

Cutting the cannabis clones isn't as simple as it sounds. In fact, it's quite technical. First of all, a farmer must identify whether the parent plant of a clone is from a male or female. The only way to tell a plant's sex is to wait until after pollination. Only then can the recognizable flowers of a female plant be seen. Pollinated female plants will produce seeds eventually and they are only needed for replanting and have no value to the consumer.

Determining a Cannabis Plant's Sex - Method 1
Grow rooms are controlled environments and they simulate the natural growing conditions with the use of technology, as mentioned above. Before pollination, cannabis plants need around 18 hours of sunlight and around 6 hours of darkness. In grow rooms; growers adjust light settings to 12 hours light and 12 hours dark to start the pollination process. This mimics the natural conditions of the late summer, which will prompt the budding process. When the first budding signs occur, farmers will isolate the female plants and ensure that the 18-hour light and 6-hour darkness timings are set. This is to make the plants revert to the pre-budding stage. When the plants do so, then clippings of the female plant clones can begin and they

are replanted. Using this method farmers then know that the future plants will all be female.

Method 2

Another way to get the female clones is by randomly cutting clones before the plants are going to bud then replanting them and allowing the parent plants to bud. All clones should be carefully marked for easy identification so the growers know which plant they came from originally.

When the parent plants bud and they are female, the clones, which were taken from them, can be confirmed as female cannabis plants. Then, female clones will be separated (they wouldn't have reached any significant stage of maturity) and groomed so they can continue growing until maturity.

If it is found that a parent plant is a male, then clones from it will be destroyed thus saving growers time and effort in growing them.

CHAPTER 8: THE GROWTH CYCLE

The growth cycle of a cannabis plant will depend on whether the plant is grown indoors or out. For example, plants grown in grow rooms will take around eleven or twelve weeks before the cannabis seedlings grow to fully mature plants for harvesting. In some cases, growers can stretch the cycle for up to six or even eight months.

The growth cycle could take a bit longer if the plants are cultivated outdoors due to environmental conditions like light and other environmental factors which cannot be controlled. There are more advanced growing methods such as aeroponics and hydroponics that will take a shorter period because nutrition and water are supplied directly to the plants, as is light.

Growth cycles may be longer or shorter for several reasons. It could be the cannabis strain itself, the height that a grower wants the plants to be, and the length of time plants are left in the flowering state before being harvested. Certain other factors that relate to how they are grown come into it too. For example, grow mediums, fertilizer types, lighting conditions as well as other circumstances.

It takes between one to four weeks to set up equipment for a grow room and order the seeds and the clones. This is the time that growers, especially first-timers, should factor in. Using clones is a time saver for growers and will shorten the actual growing period.

Seedling

This will take between 2 to 6 weeks at temperatures of 70 to 85°F. The photoperiod is 18 hours of light and 6 hours of darkness. Generally, clones or seeds are planted in smaller pots or other blocks of growing mediums. Seedlings will start to establish enough roots and also leaves, which will allow them to then move onto the vegetative state.

Most seedlings will grow enough in four to six weeks so they can be transplanted into bigger pots where they continue to grow until they can be harvested. Bigger pots will have more space so the roots can grow and also modify. Grow pots must have holes at the bottom so that excess water can drain off.

The Vegetative Stage

This takes around 2 to 6 weeks with temperatures above – 70-85°F and 18 hours of light with 6 hours of darkness. This stage can last from 2 weeks to around 2 months. The growers will decide how long or short it will take. In some cases, growers prefer tall plants for harvesting bigger buds, and in others cases, growers prefer to harvest the plants quickly and then begin growing new batches. They would not allow the plants to exceed a two to three week vegetative state.

The plants will require a fertilizer with a high nitrogen content during the vegetative stage. This will be necessary after two to three watering periods.

Flowering, Budding and Blooming
This stage takes between eight to twelve weeks at the same temperatures as above with 12 hours of light and 12 hours of darkness for 6 weeks to 4 months. This is the stage where the flowers will become dense then form buds on the branches. It is at this stage that the leaves will be coated with the resins that contain tetrahydrocannabinol. The Sativa strains will take longer than the Indica species.

Using fertilizers with high phosphorous levels is applied during the cannabis plant's flowering stage. The fertilizer should be applied at the same rate as it is during the vegetative stage. The plants will then be ready to harvest after the flowering stage.

Harvesting

Most cannabis buds fully develop within 2 weeks during harvest. When the color of the pistils or white hairs changes to orange and brownish red, it is a clear indicator that the buds are ready to be harvested. If mature plants are left too long, mold infestation could occur.

The flowers right at the top will mature much faster than the ones at the bottom. Growers trim and cut the flowers of the cannabis plant using pruning shears. The fan leaves will be trimmed then the plants are categorized according to their particular strain, and manicured. This is done by removing any excess leaves that might be around the colas. This allows them to dry quickly.

Once they are trimmed, the buds will be either hung for drying or placed on screens in a well-ventilated, dark room. The time taken for the buds to be completely dry is between 2 to 10 days. Growers must be careful however, because sometimes the cannabis buds may seem to be dry but are still wet inside. Sometimes, growers will put the buds in a polythene bag or container and seal it, leaving it for another couple of hours so the water in the bud can redistribute. If they are still wet when they are removed then they will be hung or spread out to dry. This process is repeated until the buds are dried thoroughly. This water redistribution is called "curing" or "sweating." The buds can then be stashed in Ziploc airtight bags or compressed in some jars to be used later. They should be kept in dark, cold areas.

CHAPTER 9: HYDROPONIC CANNABIS CULTIVATION

Hydroponic farming is the latest high-tech, cutting edge platform offering growers another way to grow cannabis. It is becoming so popular, and for very good reasons. It is an efficient way of farming since it doesn't use much time or energy sucking systems like in more traditional farming methods. The space that it requires is a lot smaller and it allows for a neater and more sanitary farming method that reduces the potential for disease in a big way.

Hydroponic farming is generally low maintenance and gives farmers a lot of control. It also delivers crop yields that are reported to be 100% more than other known farming techniques. Different hydroponic systems exist, all of them mostly containing these four main elements:

1. A basin or a PVC pipe where pots that contain grow mediums are placed. They may contain mineral based pellets or fibers. The plant roots will be held in the pots. Alternatively, baskets with pellets may be utilized for some individual plants. They can be placed in the basin.
2. Water reservoirs (usually found below the basins).
3. A pump for aerating the water reservoir.

4. An efficient water cycle is created when the water is pumped into the basin and from the reservoir it is drained back into the basin.

Hydroponic systems that are more sophisticated will pump water using a timer. The regular ones will simply pump the water slowly and allow it to move across this system. An electricity generator and water pump must be made especially for a hydroponic system. These systems require water to be pumped through them at regular intervals.

The water must have the correct pH level, right temperature and fertilizer specifically for cannabis plants. The nutrients needed will change during the lifecycle of the plant and must be carefully monitored. If any changes are noticed then appropriate steps must be taken in order to curb them.

Cannabis buds that are harvested using hydroponic systems tend to be larger. Initially, a hydroponic system's operation may be a little intensive until it's understood. Once it is, it becomes much easier to implement. Less effort needs to go into hydroponic farming; however, care must be taken because plants can be quite sensitive to adverse conditions.

Hydroponic farming eliminates the need for soil or soil-less mixes which are the basic foundations of traditional farming. It will provide nutrients to the plant root directly through water as well as providing oxygen through aeration. This oxygen availability at the root level will speed up the plants' nutritional intake, which in turn will hasten the cannabis plants growth and bud production.

Cuts or clones that are grown in Rockwell cubes are more preferred for hydroponic systems because it is easy to place them in the basket, pot, or PVC pipe and they will continue to grow. Rockwell cubes contain fibers that allow the water free passage to the plant roots.

Hydroponic systems will need lighting conditions that are the same as those found in indoor cultivation mediums. The growth cycle is generally shorter and the harvesting will take place earlier.

CHAPTER 10: OUTDOOR CULTIVATION

For many centuries, cannabis was grown outdoors in nature, as are all other plants. Hydroponic systems have only recently been used. Cannabis grown outside is believed to have a stronger scent and deeper flavor as well as a better taste than cannabis grown indoors or through other methods.

The cannabis plants can grow pretty much anywhere around the world, from Asia to Alaska. Both Sativa and Indica strains adapt well to tropical and temperate climates. In the Northern Hemisphere, the outdoor growing would normally take place from April to October.

Cannabis growing outdoors is pollinated naturally. Its seeds are dispersed mostly by the wind. The seeds eventually find their way back into the soil then regrow and replenish the plant population naturally.

Farmers who engage in outdoor cannabis farming face a lot of challenges and this discourages many people from doing this unless it is their only option. No one can control nature or its environmental conditions, and security is also something else they must contend with. It is not just security from people, who might stumble upon an outdoor cannabis garden and decide to help themselves to it, but also animals who could do so and destroy the plants unintentionally. It is also a gamble if the grower lives in an area where cannabis cultivation is illegal. The threat of arrest and incarceration is there. In many countries, cannabis cultivation is not illegal and can be grown outdoors without fear of arrest.

Due to the fact that cannabis plants thrive on light, it can be a bit tricky for growers who live in temperate or colder climates. Growers living in tropical areas can grow cannabis twice a year or more but growers in temperate regions can probably only do so once during the warmer months.

The Growing Site: For those considering outdoor cultivation, a convenient and secure location must be chosen. Sometimes it can be in a back yard or a more remote place such as a forest where there will be little or no security intrusions. Growers who choose to farm in forests do so in order to hide their cultivation activities. The soil must be tested to ensure it has the right pH levels and low acidity and its proximity will determine how often growers can inspect the plants to check on their growth.

The best type of sites are those that do not have any blockage from sunlight, such as larger trees or buildings. The site must be cleared and then planting beds must be raised to at least 6 or 8 inches above the ground. Once the beds have been prepared, growers will bring compost material such as leaves and grass or vegetative matter. It will then be left to rot. Preparing sites outdoors takes time; sometimes a month or up to six months before the clones or seedlings can be prepared for planting.

Transplant of clones and seedlings: Clones or seedlings can be used even if the site's soil is tough. Watering arrangements must be made, especially in the earlier growth stages. The seedlings are often sprouted indoors. Growers will usually sprout a lot more seeds than they intend to plant because some seeds might not survive in the outdoors. It's better though to sprout the seeds in normal outdoor settings as the change from the artificial indoor lights to outdoor sunlight can be harsh for them.

For those who must sprout their seeds inside, it will be necessary to gradually acclimatize the seedlings to sunlight. They could be kept in a shaded area before being gradually introduced to direct sunlight. The white sprouts of the germinated seeds are then put into the soil about half an inch and left to grow. If transplanting clones or seedlings, it is best to do it by the middle of April with its longer days and shorter nights so the flowering stage won't be induced too early.

Sunlight: There's no controlling the light outdoors. Some growers erect light bulbs if their sites are near their homes in order to "trick" the plant into believing it is still daylight and will remain in the vegetative state for a little longer.

Water: The amount of water needed will depend on how dry the soil is when growing cannabis outdoors. Farmers will try to use sites that are located near lakes, rivers, creeks or streams. If this cannot be done then alternative water sources need to be implemented such as water tanks and a hose or an irrigation system. More water is required during the vegetative stage.

Fertilizer: The more natural, organic fertilizers such as animal droppings, bone meal, blood meal, worm castings, etc. are preferred for outdoor growing. Where these are not readily available then chemical fertilizers containing higher Nitrogen ratios to Phosphorous and Potassium ratios (5:1:1) are a great alternative. Over fertilization is avoided and fertilizers must always be used according to the guidelines. The plants have to be observed for any unusual changes during the fertilizer application period.

The Wind: Strong winds can threaten the cannabis plants outdoors but there are a couple of things that can be done to protect them from any wind damage. Firstly, other plants could be grown around them that will act as a windbreaker. The only problem with this is that the other plants will likely compete with the cannabis plants for nutrients and water. Secondly, metal or wooden stakes can be placed in the ground and the plants can be tied to them. Thirdly, the construction of a fence around the cannabis plants can be created. It can be made out of string, Velcro, trellis netting, or extendable wire and can support the cannabis plants during their different growth stages.

Pest Control & Weeding: Pests will vary outdoors and include insects (spider mites, whiteflies, mealybugs,) to animals and birds. It is when the cannabis plants are at a younger stage that the pests are more of a threat. One way to combat this is by using companion planting. This means planting stronger smelling plants such as mint, garlic, cloves, or cayenne pepper in between the cannabis. Some insects or animals such as ladybugs, frogs and birds will feed on the insect pests. Pesticides made at home using dish washing liquid and garlic extract can also be very effective. A fence can help to keep animals out.

When it comes to weeds, they must be removed frequently so the cannabis plants aren't deprived of any essential nutrients. It is better to remove the weeds manually. Weed killers will have a detrimental effect and should not be used.

Harvesting: When the pistils turn an orange-red, it is a sign that the cannabis plants are ready to be harvested. Once the buds are harvested, they can be dried outdoors, preferably under some sort of enclosure or a tent that can protect the delicate buds and dry them faster. Another way to do it is to trim the branches or pull out the plants and dry them indoors.

In some cases, growers will leave the male plants to flower then pollinate the female plants and produce seeds they can then replant. The trick is to know when to pull out the plants – not too early. The bracts or sheaths are opened so growers can check for the brown color that lets them know if the plants are ready to be harvested or not.

CONCLUSION

As you can see, cannabis is a versatile and useful plant and history has shown us that this is indeed true. Cannabis has been cultivated for thousands of years throughout human history, and this continues today.

Whatever method is chosen to cultivate cannabis, they will all be unique and have their own advantages. Every grower is different too so they will choose the method that suits them. Farmers are continually researching better ways of growing cannabis and improving their methods to produce higher crop yields and better quality harvests.

There is a lot of information on cannabis growing and cannabis in general that you can research for yourself. It is available at your local library and indeed, at your fingertips through the Internet. Numerous cannabis websites and blogs exist and are there for people to gain even more information. Local farmers are also a valuable source of information, and their challenges and techniques will add another dimension to your knowledge. Your local farmers will have information that is particular to the area in which you live.

Just another reminder to make sure you make yourself familiar and comply with the laws in your particular area regarding cannabis cultivation and use before embarking on any cannabis project. Cannabis use or cultivation that is illegal will pose great risks to the individual.

It can be exciting and also rewarding to grow your own cannabis. The whole process will become easier the more it is practiced and you gain more experience.

THANKS FOR READING

We really hope you enjoyed this book. If you found this material helpful feel free to share it with friends. You can also help others find it by leaving a review where you purchased the book. Your feedback will help us continue to write books you love.

The Smart Reads library is growing by the day! Make sure and check out the other wonderful books in our catalog. We would love to hear which books are your favorite.

SMART READS ORIGINS

Smart Reads was born out of the desire to find the best information fast without having to wade through the sheer volume of fluff available online. Smart Reads combs through massive amounts of knowledge compiles the best into quick to read books on a variety of subjects.

We consider ourselves Smart Readers, not dummies. We know reading is smart. We're self taught. We like to learn a TON about a WIDE variety of topics. We have developed a love for books and we find intelligence attractive.

We found that each new topic we tried to learn about started with the challenge of finding the pieces of the puzzle that mattered most. It becomes a treasure hunt rather than an education.

Smart Reads wants to find the best of the best information for you. To condense it into a package that you can consume in an hour or less. So you can read more books about more topics in less time.

OUR MISSION

Smart Reads aims to accelerate the availability of useful information and will publish a high quality book on every major topic on amazon.

Smart Reads hopes to remove barriers to sharing by taking the copyright off everything we publish and donating it to the public domain. We hope other publishers and authors will follow our example.

Our goal is to donate $1,000,000 or more by 2020 to build over 2,000 schools by giving 5% of our net profit to Pencils of Promise.

We want to restore forests around the globe by planting a tree for every 10 physical books we sell and hope to plant over 100,000 trees by 2020.

Doesn't it feel good knowing that by educating yourself you are helping the world be a better place? We think so too...

Thanks for helping us help the world. You Smart Reader you...

Travis and the Smart Reads Team

WHY I STARTED SMART READS

Every time I wanted to learn about something new I'd have to buy 20 books on the topic and spend way too long sorting through them and reading them all until I arrived at the big picture. Until I had enough perspectives to know who was just guessing, who was uninformed and who had stumbled upon something remarkable.

I wished someone else could just go in and figure that out for me and tell me what matters. That's how smart reads was born. I want smart reads to be a company that does all that research up front. Sorts through all the content that is available on each topic and pulls out the most up to date complete understanding, then have people smarter than me package the best wisdom in an easy to understand way in the least amount of words possible.

For example, I got a new puppy so I wanted to learn about dog training. I bought 14 different books about dog training and by the time I got through the first 5 and finally started getting the big picture on the best way to train my puppy she had grown up into a dog.

Yeah she's well behaved. She doesn't poop in the house. I can get her to sit and come when I call. But what if someone else went in and read all those books for me, found the underlying themes and picked out the best information that would give me the big picture and get me right to the point. And I'd only have to read one book instead of 15.

That would be amazing. I would save time. And maybe my dog would be rolling over, cleaning up after my kids and doing the dishes by now. That my friend, is the reason I started smart reads. Because I wanted a company I can trust to deliver me the best information in an easy to understand way that I can digest in under an hour. Because dog training is one of many subjects I want to master.

The quicker I can learn a wide variety of topics the sooner that information can begin playing a role in shaping my future. And none of us knows how long that future will be. So why not do everything we can to make the best of it and consume a ton of knowledge. And I figured all the better if I can also make a positive difference in the world.

That's why we're also building schools, planting trees and challenging ideas about copyright's place in today's world. Because as a company we have to be doing everything we can to support the ecosystem that gives us all these beautiful places to read our books. Thanks for reading.

Travis

Customers Who Bought This Customers Who Bought This Book Also Bought

The Cannabis Pharmacy: Grow Cannabis, Make Hemp Oil and Know the Difference Between THC, CBD and the Medical Benefits of Cannabinoids

?

Mint As Medicine: Discover The Powerful Healing Properties of Herb in Treating Headaches, Allergies, Asthma, Clarity and Peace of Mind

The Powerful Benefits of Myrrh: Effective Myrrh Recipes For Healthy & Beauty, Oil Pulling Therapy, Creativity, Aromatherapy and Improving The Mind

Beginner Gardening: Growing Vegetables and Ornamentals

Epsom Salt: Holistic Recipes for Beautiful Skin, Pain Relief and Relaxation

Natural Ways of Boosting Testosterone: How to Bulk Up and Put Your Sex Drive in Overdrive

MDMA and Other Psychedelic Drugs: Learning the Therapeutic Effects of LSD, Psilocybin and Other Mind-Bending Drugs